A PHYSICIAN'S GUIDE TO THE STUDY
OF THE NON-LINEAR MIND
KELEE® MEDICINE

A PHYSICIAN'S GUIDE TO THE STUDY OF THE NON-LINEAR MIND KELEE® MEDICINE

Learning to Heal with Compassion

Amy M. Sitapati, MD[1]

Introduction by Ron W Rathbun[2]

A PHYSICIAN'S GUIDE TO THE STUDY
OF THE NON-LINEAR MIND
KELEE® MEDICINE

This book is an original publication of the Kelee® Foundation

PRINTING HISTORY
first edition / December 2019

www.thekelee.org
ISBN: 978-0-9841608-7-7

PRINTED IN THE UNITED STATES OF AMERICA

Acknowledgements

Heartfelt thanks for the friendship, suggestions, and recommendations from Ron W Rathbun[2], Dan Lee, MD[1], Frank Silva, Ankita Kadakia, MD[1], Sanjeev Bhavnani, MD[3], Louis Sands, Nikki Walsh, MBA, and D'Arcy Harley, MSW. The experience of this dynamic team is beyond words. (1) UC San Diego, (2) Kelee Foundation, and (3) Scripps Clinic. *Their collective contribution to Kelee Medicine is beyond words.*

*The feeling in your mind fuels
the feeling in your body.
When your mind
is growing and learning,
it is that feeling
that manifests health and healing*[2].

Table of Contents

_____

There are only two things
in the universe,
you and everything else.
It would be wise,
to understand these two places
in your mind[2].

Definitions

Kelee® Medicine: learning to heal with the non-linear harmonious energy of mind.

Empathy: is a mind-body attached energy within us all that connects consciousness and chemistry.

Self-Compassion: is the understanding of our own pain.

Compassion: is the understanding of another's pain, without the taking on of another's pain.

Linear Mind: is a mind that uses another (reflection) point to learn.

Non-Linear Mind: is a mind that understands directly without a biased second point.

One-Pointed Process: the non-linear ability—in mind to observe, without a second point of comparison to understand, thus eliminating biased analysis.

Two-Pointed Process: a process of mind, that uses two points of comparison to learn.

Detachment: the ability to not be distracted or controlled by a second point.

Attachment: when a second point adversely affects the primary point of mind.

Non-Interference: to not intimidate or coerce a person, to alter or change their natural course of action in life.

———————————

Teach those ...
who want to learn,
heal those
who want to be healed,
and all others
will heal in time[2].

Introduction

– Ron W. Rathbun

I have been working with MDs since 1995, and a common problem arises with them. How do I not be so affected by my patients? They feel empathy for their patients and then are affected by them. Addressing this problem was a major focus in my work, of understanding the mind and Kelee meditation. Finding a concise way to show people how to free themselves from unhealthy influence. This is what I came to understand.

Most people in the world have felt empathy and have heard of compassion[5], at one time or another. What people don't know about empathy and compassion is that they are part of the same, non-linear energy within us all. What connects the mental and physical parts of our being is, empathy, it is an attached energy that connects our heart, with our head. Empathy is a mind—body attached energy that connects consciousness and chemistry. Empathy is an energy of caring, which is necessary and healthy for us, however, when we care too much about others and it affects us, it becomes our problem.

Empathy is a non-linear energy, based in mental feeling, not in linear thinking. The energy of empathy resides in the lesser Kelee[4] (LK) and greater Kelee[4] (GK). Empathy connects and binds the LK and GK together. It is hard wired into our instinctual process of living. Empathy is strong in the parental part of life in women for nurturing, and in men, it stimulates protection instincts. This is also why people struggle to understand it, because of its non-linear nature.

When people are too empathetic with others, they will want to be close to another and put themselves in an unhealthy state of mind, that can affect their health. When we feel empathy for someone hurting, we tend to connect our energy to them, by forming an attachment[5]. We drop our energy level to be with them, at their level. This is not good for us, because we have now allowed ourselves to become attached to them and allowed ourselves to feel their mental and physiological pain, which begins to then affect us. If you, now feel bad, how can you help another? Now you can begin to loop through them and your interaction with them has become unhealthy for you. So how do you stop this from happening? How do you deal with what feels so natural, but is so hard to control? We must learn some mental skills called the art of detachment[5].

(4) Basic Principles of the Kelee defined in back of book.
(5) See definitions in the front of the book.

We must learn the difference, between the attached energy of empathy, and the detached energy of self-compassion[5]. We must learn how to open, and use the non-attached energy of the mind, only then, can we be open with someone hurting, and be unaffected by them. When our vibratory rate is harmonious, we are in a place to help others. When we are in a disharmonious space, we are not.

It is when we learn self-compassion, the understanding of our own pain, that we can understand another's, and not be affected by them. Self-compassion has a counterpart, which is compassion, the ability to be harmonious within oneself, and helpful in a world filled with pain and suffering. Compassion is an energy that others can feel, and when you feel it within, others can feel it from you, if they are open. Once people learn to open their mind through Kelee meditation, they can open to self-compassion, then they can also learn how to open to the beautiful energy of compassion and be an example of how each of us can help our fellow human beings.

– *Ron W. Rathbun*
Founder of the Kelee

Being one pointed ...
and still of mind,
is the purest non distracted place
you will ever experience.
It is also a state of mind,
that is
complete freedom [2].

Foreword

Physicians are drawn to heal. The practice of Kelee meditation offers an opportunity to bring mind and body into a harmonious balance. The application of this practice begins with self-understanding. As a result of the practice of Kelee meditation, you will discover the benefits of mental stillness. This results in detachment from that which hurts you. As you detach from compartments[4] that are a source of dysfunction, you will discover self-compassion and mental strength. The non-linear mind[5] then becomes the source of self-healing. The Anatomy of the Kelee and the Basic Principles of the Kelee provide the structural framework for self-understanding. This text serves as a field guide for physicians seeking balance and healing for themselves and their patients. Here, we provide experiences, insights, anatomical reference points, and concepts through Kelee meditation, which can help you bring balance to mind and body. The harmony of non-linear mind results in self-healing, which can be shared with others. This is known as Kelee Medicine[5].

Keywords: Kelee meditation, Meditation, Medicine, Non-linear mind, Self-Compassion, Compassion

(4) Basic Principles of the Kelee defined in back of book.
(5) See definitions in the front of the book.

_____

Learning to heal
with
compassion[1].

A Physician's Guide to the Study of the Non-Linear Mind Kelee Medicine

Why study the non-linear mind in medicine?
We have all been there.

Young, bright, and inspired to make a difference in the world; we entered the profession. We completed our training with endless hours of study, clinical rotations, and sleepless nights in the hopes of improving medicine. Now, practicing our art, we heal our patients, the afflicted. Yet, somehow, in the journey, our personal humanness and grounding can become lost. Feeling like a ship lost at sea without our sextant, we can lose sight of how to help improve the wellness of our patients and ourselves.

This simple field guide serves to provide stories and structure to help you better understand the important role of the non-linear mind in the practice of medicine. The ten lessons shared are intended to be for physicians to apply in their professional and personal lives. The structure of each lesson includes reflection, clinical context, and the Basic Principles of the Kelee. In the last chapter, a few reflections about Kelee Medicine from conversations with practicing physicians and close friends are shared in the form of questions and answers related to burnout and healing.

*Into the depths
of the greater Kelee,
I dropped.
The nectar of healing[1].*

Lesson 1:
Discovery of Compassion
and Healing

A physician's life is drawn from earnest desire to ease the suffering of another through compassion, intellect, and action. The path is distinct. To effectively heal, the patient must trust, try, and receive healing for themselves. We, alongside our patients, are exposed to a variety of physical, emotional, mental, and spiritual challenges.

As a result, we may attach to our patients and experience their pain. We feel a change in our energy, balance, and well-being. When we attach to a patient's disharmony we experience depletion in our energy as a result of empathy. Empathy is the result of taking on the pain and dysfunction of another at your own expense. This comes in the form of experiencing fear, pain, and suffering resulting in loss of energy and loss of harmony.

The following explains the difference between empathy and compassion. A physician begins the visit with a full cup of energy, and the patient is with less than 1/4 cup of energy. The physician interacts with the patient through empathy and feels the patient's pain. Following the visit, not only has the physician lost energy with only 1/2 cup of energy left for the day but also the patient, leaves in no better state still with less than 1/4 cup of energy. Empathy is a two-pointed[5] process that results in a loss of energy, from the physician.

Compare this interaction to compassion. The physician meets the same patient with less than 1/4 cup of energy. The physician shares compassion and remains one-pointed in their greater Kelee. As a result, the physician does not lose any energy. Further, the patient leaves feeling better with a rise in energy represented by a cup that is now 1/2 full.

You may ask, "how do you experience the difference between empathy and compassion in a clinical setting?" Why does empathy result in a loss of energy? To better understand this, let us consider Jenny, a 42-year old landscaper, who lost her mother in March. She has elevated blood pressure (BP) and troubled sleep. As she begins to share what is going on in her life, she tears up and shares exasperation.

With empathy, you feel her pain. In fact, as she shares her loss, you cry and become heavy-hearted. You offer condolences, medication to help sleep, counseling and a follow up in two weeks. You are spent and feel tired as you leave the room, and Jenny was the first of 18 patients

(5) See definitions in the front of the book.

of the day! How did this happen? You accepted the disharmonious energy from Jenny, and this resulted in you accepting her pain as your own. While this may have seemed to help, she left feeling empty. The exchange came at your expense and left you feeling low.

Compassion is different. Compassion is about the understanding of Jenny's pain but not taking on the disharmonious feeling as your own. When you are able to stay one-pointed in the non-linear mind, you can listen to Jenny, have understanding, and thereby have compassion, but not compromise the way you feel on the inside. Jenny, will often, in fact, feel the harmony that you have from within, and accept this herself as hers. In fact, as Jenny leaves the office, she may feel better. This is a form of healing from non-linear mind.

Still deep night black.
Nothing. Empty.
The mind blank.

Lesson 2:
Self-Awareness
A Key to Well-Being

In order for you to maintain well-being and balance, we physicians must first look to care for ourselves and understand our own mind. Basic physician wellness begins with self-care, both physically and mentally. From a physical perspective, are you getting adequate rest, sleep, exercise, and nutrition? On the mental side, do you have peace of mind free from stress and negative thoughts? Are you able to achieve mental stillness? Have you taken time to look in your mind and as a result, foster self-awareness?

The first step in this journey is to discover your conscious awareness. Right now, your awareness is focused on this text at the second point outside of 'you' on this page. By practicing Kelee meditation, you can learn to direct your awareness to a primary point within you or a secondary point outside of you. Primary point is the non-linear mind that is inside you. Secondary point is everything else. This can include focus outside you, on an object or a person. It can also include a focus on your breath or heartbeat by physical feeling of your body. Being in control of your conscious awareness means that you must first be able to sense your conscious awareness. This comes as a result of detaching from what hurts you.

Compartments are misunderstandings that exist in your Kelee that you hold on to. Compartments represent everything that remains unresolved in your mind that hurts you. For most of us, what remains unresolved in our mind we don't want to look at because we either do not understand it or associate it with negative feelings. However, compartments accumulate over time. If you pay attention, compartments have an unresolved thought and a negative feeling. This unresolved thought then influences the experience that you and your patient have.

Take, for example, John, your second patient of the morning, who greets you as the door opens with a scowl and a phrase, "This office is a disgrace! You should be embarrassed to work in such a place!" John is far from being in a good space. Admittedly, his 60-hour workweek and his negative feeling that his job is dead-end are not helping. Yet, as the physician entering the room, you may find that you are feeling fear-based brain chatter. "What if he accuses me of something? What if he makes me feel bad?" Internally, you may have brain chatter that results in distraction. As a result, you may continue to have negative chatter even after leaving the room. Subsequently, you may not even be aware that you need to use the restroom or take a quick break for a drink of water.

You may wear the feeling of fear and negativity as you enter the room of patient three, Marion, who was diagnosed with metastatic renal cell cancer last month. She senses the fear that you have and is also triggered by her fear of mortality. By the end of the workday, you may feel exhausted both physically and emotionally.

As physicians, we are pulled many directions with multiple competing priorities. Early in our careers, we learn and are celebrated for our stamina. Stay up all night in the intensive care unit (ICU) with a ventilated patient whose pulse is 140, and oxygen saturation last 87% on 100% fraction of inspired oxygen (FiO_2). Stand in the operating room (OR) for 15 hours [without food, water, and restroom breaks] in a complicated open-heart surgery. We are trained and encouraged to have a form of stamina that helps us complete tasks at our own expense.

While on an individual occurrence basis, this may not serve the patient's interests on a day in and day out, week by week basis. By practicing Kelee meditation, one can improve mental stillness and as a result, have an improved awareness of our needs and the needs of our patients. This mental strength also provides us with the ability to better balance the physical and mental needs that we have as a result of being human. Our mental strength will provide us with a better ability over the long haul to ensure that we maintain physiological balance and clarity of mind, two characteristics that will be essential for our well-being.

_The difference
between
pushing and
walking alongside_.

Lesson 3:
Non-Interference and
Cessation of Looping

Perhaps one of the most difficult concepts for a maturing physician is non-interference[5]. We are trained to take control of poor health, dysfunction, biology, and chemistry imbalance. We are trained to interrupt and reverse health decline.

We have all been taught to interfere. We learn algorithms that "check and mate" our patients with their behaviors. Perhaps you can remember a time when you chided someone for smoking, mandated adherence [if you don't --, then --!], and so on. Was the patient open when they left that day? Were they engaged and looking forward to following your recommendation? Or, did the patient then suffer with mental chatter belittled with guilt and self-doubt? We should all do well to delicately balance our recommendations to be congruent with patient self-understanding.

The intersection between healing as a physician and interference is certainly a delicate one. As a patient in need shares a visit with us, we try to define a course of action. Is it congruent with what the patient wants? Does it fulfill what the patient is seeking, or rather is this for the physician to 'improve', 'fix', and 'win'! Are you meeting the patient at their readiness, or are you ascribing an agenda of your own accord? What are the underpinning drivers of action for you

(5) See definitions in the front of the book.

and your patient? Does peer acceptance and fear play a role in your advisement?

Marcus is a 65-year old architect who carries a busy lifestyle and has long commutes to work. He presents with a body mass index (BMI) 37 kg/m^2, a systolic blood pressure (SBP) 147 mm Hg, and fingerstick glucose (FSG) 131. He is relatively happy with life and wants to know what his health status is. Should you?

(a) Share the newest research on diet and exercise, and tell him to institute it right away.

(b) Detail patient-oriented goals over 30 minutes that includes exercise, low carbohydrate, and low salt diet, and follow up in one month.

(c) Refer the patient to a nutritionist and advise that he also get a gym membership.

(d) Inform the patient that weight, BP, and glucose are up. Ask the patient whether he might want to return in three months to further discuss his plan to address health.

What do you believe is the most common approach that we are trained as physicians to use? And, which options have less interference? What is interference anyways? Interference is the act of imparting a thought or feeling on another. This is often a result of looping[4] between two people. Individual looping is when an unresolved thought and disharmonious feeling, as a result of a compartment being triggered, circle unresolved leading to mental chatter.

(4) Basic Principles of the Kelee defined in back of book.

Two people can also loop with each other. In the physician practice, interference can result in looping between physician and patient. For example, Dr. Smith, in an effort to aid his patients to change their health behaviors, has developed a control algorithm related to diabetic diet healthy behaviors. Dr. Smith's algorithm is 'patients with diabetes should never eat sugar.'

Then the patient, Betsy, arrives at the clinic. Betsy has Type II diabetes with a glycated HbA1C that has been creeping up to 8.5. Betsy is stressed with a recent breakup and has been eating M&M'S® to cope. Dr. Smith scolds Betsy, "You know better, your HbA1C is up because you are unable to stick to the diet. No sugar, Betsy. This is an absolute!" Then, Betsy answers back to the physician, "You are right, I know better. I am so sorry, Dr. Smith." Betsy continues to be triggered, and mental chatter follows, "I am the worst! Why do I always do such a terrible job in my life. I really suck!" As Betsy, walks to her car after the visit, she is still with mental chatter and is looping with herself. Inside, she is thinking, "I will never be good enough, I can't even keep myself from eating M&M'S. No one will ever love me!"

As you can see, physicians tread a fine line in offering counseling and support but not at the patient's expense. Physicians should rather learn to be still in one-pointed mind. Patients can sense one-pointed mind in their physician, and may choose to accept a feeling of understanding, compassion, and love.

There is a subtlety
beyond words
at the still point,
quiet and soft[1]*.*

Lesson 4:
Non-Linear
Inspiration to Heal

Was there a day that you recall your inspiration to further bring healing into the world? We all have stories of our individual and unique journeys to heal. Mine was at age 17, and her name was "Tonya". Volunteering at the local children's hospital and finding myself assigned to befriend an individual living a far different life experience than my own, I met Tonya.

Tonya had been afflicted with cystic fibrosis, and increasingly found breathing more labored and tiresome. She was spending as much time on the pediatric inpatient unit as in her home and hence was seeking to find friendship from a companion her age. I knew nothing of charts, doctors, and the practice of medicine, but I could tell by how she moved that at some point in the not too distant future, she might not walk out of the hospital's doors.

Nevertheless, I humbly accepted the assignment eager to lend a hand, ear, and heart. We met regularly once or twice

_When you are inspired
to find,
you most assuredly will_[2].

a week, sometimes just quietly sharing the room and other times eager to discuss crafts, the world, and her #1 sport adoration—football.

Over time I learned that medicine had optimized what it could of her plight, and she was seeking a 'friend' during her journey that connected with her 'youth'. I came to enjoy our conversations and wheeling her around the hospital. I also appreciated the great lengths that her medical treatment team made to extend her life. My mind was inspired to help in healing and bring comfort to those like "Tonya".

It is from this inspiration that my journey was chartered. What about you? From our deepest selves, non-linear mind, we find who we are. We connect to the purpose that seeded what we do today. Perhaps, you, like me, are inspired from the heart to help ease suffering, discover purpose among health challenge, and just connect deeply to those that we care for. Inspired from the inside to practice this art, we call medicine.

———————————

*It just didn't
feel right,
and that
was enough.*

Lesson 5:
Seeing from Stillness of Mind
Clearly

As we assemble information, we take note of movement, expression, physical findings, laboratory values, and so on. We aim to master the diagnosis and treatment plan. Increasingly, our evidence-based medicine has fostered the algorithm of treatment.

Certainly, this has dramatically furthered our understanding of the role of particular therapeutics in modifying the pathophysiology of our patients. Yet, sometimes, we just have an innate feeling that we have 'gotten it all wrong!' It comes down to the sense that we can't put our finger on, a suspicion, a reason, not to trust option 'A' as the right answer. We feel pulled inside to look for something else, break the algorithm, and do something different for the patient in front of us. This is our 'gut' instinct.

I remember the very first instance as a physician in training that I anchored this knowing. I had scrubbed into a gynecological-oncology case. The patient on the table was being prepped for a laparoscopic incision. Everything looked fine—experienced surgeon, several surgical residents at the elbow, an experienced anesthesiologist. The patient was unconscious by now, and vitals all fine. I got a cramp in my stomach, so to speak. I looked down the table as a fourth-year medical student and could not shake the feeling that the seasoned surgeon was about to perforate the inferior epigastric artery as the trocar entered the abdomen.

It was a feeling first, unsettling. Should I say something? Then, my brain next went, 'this surgeon has more than 20 years of experience, there is no way that they would make such an error.' Decision - 'say nothing, you are a mere medical student!' That is when it happened, in the snap of a finger, blood squirting everywhere and all hands on the abdomen. The subsequent 20 minutes were consumed in tying off the bleeding and starting over again. That is when I discovered the mind of a physician is as important as the brain.

This is an example of seeing clearly. It is less important to know what exactly your perception has identified as an incongruence, and more importantly, to trust the feeling that you have. Learning to 'see clearly' what you feel first and what you think second is an important skill for all physicians. This perception comes from a still mind and should not be discarded. Physicians have a refined ability to read situations at hand. If the time is not right, it is not right. You should honor what you feel. At times this may come from assimilated knowledge from thousands of observations that cannot be distilled into a simple algorithm or it may be purely from the sensitivity of your non-linear mind. Nevertheless, this sense is worth its weight in gold. Trust what you feel and see clearly!

————————————————

*Free
from compartments,
I hear more
than
what is said[2].*

Lesson 6:
Listening from Mind
Without Distraction

Learning to listen, really listen, is trusting the heart and not the ears. We have been trained to practice medicine in a methodical way. The Subjective, Objective, Assesment and Plan (SOAP) structure has brought an incredible ability to compile and share patient information with other providers and identify progression over time. However, this algorithm for documentation should not supplant what we feel. We should look to the subjective response of a patient to be both objective 'what is stated' and subjective 'what we feel'.

Johnny was 51 and life had been anything but easy. Years of drug use, smoking, and living in the streets had caught up with him and it showed on his weathered body. One night, lying down in a puddle of water, he dozed into a deep drunken slumber. As he was found the next morning on the sidewalk hypothermic, he was rushed by ambulance to the hospital. The overnight admitting team was signing him out in the morning. "Yeah, he is a real troublemaker,

_Detachment
defines a
truly open mind_[2].

that one, begging for pain medicine, a real addict." I walked into the room and immediately felt it… 'panic'.

Something was wrong. I shed the sign-out like a jacket and approached Johnny. He was near trembling. I could not wrap my head around it, 'what was this tough guy afraid of?' I then spoke, "what is wrong?" Johnny then blurted out, "it's my feet, doc, my feet, they feel like someone is cutting them off." I next looked to my team and asked, "what did your exam of the feet show?" and the response followed, "oh, I don't think that we looked." I pulled back the sheet, and to my dismay, in the spring, in temperate San Diego, there it was crisp and clear—10 necrotic black toes. Surprisingly, Johnny had frostbite, and as the next month would prove, as those toes nearly took his life, and not just his legs, he was right to be afraid.

What had happened? The treating team had triggered a previously installed compartment—patients with injection drug use history are drug seekers. They will try to get pain medications, and their demands for this should be discarded. This compartment had distracted the admitting team from looking more carefully at the patient in front of them. In mind, it could be understood that the patient was actually feeling fear. With an open mind, the underlying context could be found.

—————————

Perfection
is not
the cornerstone
of the
art of medicine.

Lesson 7:
The Mistake and
Self-Compassion

Self-compassion is one of the most important skills to learn as a healer. Doctoring is high volume, fast-paced, and complex. Increasingly, this complexity is expanding as patients survive with multi-morbidity, and knowledge grows more than ½ million publications each year! Regrets can be a commonplace, both in subtle and overt ways.

The prescription. Nearly five years ago, I remember writing the script. It was a busy day, and between patients, my nurse popped into the room and asked, "Hey, can you write a script for Jenny Someone? She says that she has a urinary tract infection (UTI) and that she dropped off a urine yesterday." Between patients, I clicked into her chart, yes, UTI, I can see that. A few clicks, and then the order was sent, amoxicillin. About one hour later, my nurse returned, "Did you really mean to send over 30 pills, the script said three times per day for seven days, didn't you mean 21 pills?" I racked my brain, how had that happened? And then I

The ability
to see clearly
brings confidence[2].

clicked into the chart and saw, 'autocompleted of quantity' by the computer. I had missed this and signed without manually entering an override.

There it was and you can see that I have still held onto it, 'the mistake'. We, doctors, have an intolerance for imperfection. Yet, working with systems and people, mistakes will happen. We can adopt a drive to create systems, people, and processes that support our abilities to provide high quality and reliable care.

Nevertheless, at the end of the day, failures are likely to continue to happen periodically. On the inside, what we need is self-compassion. The love for our skill and work that doing our best and learning from our errors is quite important. However, we cannot take all things to heart and should show ourselves self-compassion as well. This is likely the most difficult skill that you will mature as a physician and should be rendered with love and patience.

Be yourself.

Lesson 8:
Self-Acceptance
Learning to Be Yourself First

Self-acceptance is likely a trait that we believe we have garnished but can further deepen with Kelee meditation. Self-acceptance is the acceptance of you as you are, right here, right now. Many of us have been taught to accept the version of what we should be, above being ourselves. We speak in a particular way, dress in a specific way, write as we have been instructed, and so on. But, we are not robots, we are humans, with feelings. We experience our careers in a richer fashion when we bring ourselves to our practice.

Don was 45 years old and was now working 70-80 hours a week. At some point, one just loses count. And, there were lots of requirements in the job, as an academic physician, that resulted in the expansion of time commitments. It started with growing a patient practice, then added one with teaching a resident or two, then a fellow, then writing a manuscript, then joining a committee, and just rinse and repeat about 50 times.

A relaxed state
of mind
opens your
perception to
self-understanding[2].

This expansion of commitments was not logical. Also, each domain seemed intriguing but sequentially at the cost of personal time and self-expression. Running from patient to patient, trainee to trainee, committee to committee, and then iterative rewriting of manuscripts left little time. There was no time to slow down, feel self, and accept the inner self. Don's inner self wanted to wear pink socks to work, play Bob Marley in the office, and develop a training guide for the early recognition of dementia. Don had long given up his connection to self, rushing to complete the next task at hand.

Self-acceptance is deep and rich. At its core, self-acceptance allows us to be who we are. It provides us with the permission to bring ourselves to work. And, it results in our own rich and personal self-expression as we walk as healers.

Winning
is not the aim,
being present
is[1].

Lesson 9:
Accept Defeat
Winning is Not Everything

Physicians are trained winners from birth or close thereafter. We are generally selected from the educational system to be on top—winners in our classes through kindergarten onwards. We are rewarded and celebrated for being number one. We don't even have our application reviewed by the medical school, in general, unless our marks are cream of the crop. Yet, in medicine, we lose and that is common.

Marcus did everything right, but it just had not been enough. At the age of 35, the fungal infection that he had contracted was impossible to clear. Every medicine had been tried, oral, intravenous, and multiple rounds both inpatient and out. His AIDS-causing virus had been curtailed but the opportunistic infection was not showing defeat.

In spite of spinal taps, prednisone tapers to reduce cerebral edema nothing was working; he was getting worse. And then, the call came one day, "Marcus isn't coming into the clinic today, he can't get out of bed." My nurse and I looked across from each other, we could stay late and move one patient, and perhaps get across the border and back. When we showed up at his house, we ran up the narrow winding stairs. He lay there awake, staring. He motioned for the cup lying beside the bed, and his partner held his head up as he choked down about 15 tablets and capsules. I thought, 'what now?' He was grey and did not look good. I shared the report, "Yes, your viral load is doing great, still undetectable, and your CD4 is creeping up."

This fight had been going on for two years. When we first met, his pulse had been non-palpable. Following the ICU course and hospitalizations (and there were several), the situation was not looking good. Rife with a desert yeast infection when he had no immunity, our combat, including antiviral therapy, had resulted in brain swelling and a gentle rise in his CD4 cells.

This delicate balance was being fought with handfuls of medication, but after two years, Marcus was tired. He could no longer cross the border. Marcus taught me medicine beyond words. I had grown to accept defeat with a calm, caring, and loving respect. That was the last time I saw him. I will forever remember how he faced an early death, quietly persistent, calm, committed, and determined to live up to his last breath, fearless.

As physicians, we do not win 'life'. We certainly have

tools that frequently extend the quantity and or quality of life. Our skilled hands, keen eye, and trained knowledge offer opportunity to further expand the possibilities of health. That being said, our most valuable skill is our presence. We bring an inclusiveness that allows for the life cycle of humanity when we can settle and be present, regardless of the outcome.

One day at a time,
we build
the courage,
mental strength,
and love to continue
in the practice
of our art[1].

Lesson 10:
Sharing the Roots of Burnout and the Discovery of Healing

Question & Answer

While sitting with good friends including, Dr. Anita Gaind, a seasoned internist, Dr. Barbara Berkovich, a clinical informaticist instructor, and small business owner, and Dr. Lucy Savitz, a leading researcher as Vice President of Health Research at Kaiser Permanente Northwest, served as the foundation for this chapter. We shared a series of discussions about the root cause of physician burnout and how to better address physician wellness.

I have adapted the spirit of those conversations in a question and answer format below as Anita, Barbara, and Lucy provoked me to look deeper in myself. I learned that in order to understand the origins of physician burnout, we should look inside ourselves and see clearly. My dear friends and colleagues, Dan Lee, MD, Frank Silva, Ankita Kadakia, MD, Sanjeev Bhavnani, MD, and Ron W Rathbun, also contributed insightful content through their understanding.

Q: When asked recently whether I liked being a physician?

A: I answered, "Yes, I do! But, I sometimes don't like how I feel."

Q: So, why don't you feel good sometimes?

A: "I am tired."

Q: Why are you tired?

A: "There is a lot of paperwork, typing, prescriptions, phone calls, and other work to get done."

Q: Why is there so much work to be done and why are you tired? You used to stay up as a resident for days!

A: "I may work 13 hours taking care of 100 patients, including face to face visits and inbox work. Patients arrive late and hold up the scheduled ones who get irritated. My nurse gets behind, as there is no time for electrocardiograms and injections. By the end of the day, the automated lights have switched off while patients are still in the office, and there is no time for bathroom breaks, lunch, or laughter. The work is very wash, rinse, and repeat with days, weeks, and years passing in this cycle."

Q: So, is that why you feel burned out?

A: "No."

Q: Then, what do you feel is really the cause?

A: "I went into doctoring to connect with people and help them feel better."

Q: Do you feel that you connect with people now?

A: "Yes and no. I discovered that I can connect better with myself and find self-compassion. With a mental stillness of the non-linear mind and compassion, I am better able to practice the art of medicine. Connection can be one or two pointed. One-pointed stillness is from within to self. With the practice of Kelee meditation, you learn to have one-pointed connection with self. This primary point connection helps the patient more than a second point connection because it is free from distraction and disharmony."

Q: What do you mean?

A: "A few years ago, I started practicing Kelee meditation, a simple five-minute meditation twice per day that results in improved mental clarity and detachment. Detachment refers to a still mind that is not distracted by other things. These things can, for example, be brain chatter about things I have to do or mental pain about heartache that is unresolved. In a physician's office, my brain chatter can be 'hurry up—you are two patients behind!' and heartache can be the feeling of inadequacy and not being good enough from the failure to stay on time. By detaching from brain chatter and heartache, I have improved presence in the moment and peace of mind. This allows me to stay connected with myself. Put simply Kelee meditation helps me connect better with the mission of my work."

Q: So, would you say that Kelee meditation has given you resilience?

A: "Not exactly. Let me explain. Resilience refers to a bouncing back to 'baseline'. But, in Kelee, we are not becoming resilient but rather free to evolve and be more harmonious, free from compartmentalization.

As physicians, we are seeking help when we experience tragedy, but are taught to push our feelings aside. Unresolved feelings of guilt, doubt, and fear result in the accumulation of unresolved heartache leading to compartments.

By practicing Kelee meditation five minutes twice per day, this is a more powerful tool than any self-help, power yoga, wine, or counseling. By learning from ourselves, improving our self-acceptance, and growing; we continue to evolve to be who we want to be. We are no longer bouncing back in resilience but rather springing forward in self-growth and self-understanding."

Q: How do you feel that this practice has changed the way that you interact with patients?

A: "Kelee meditation has helped me improve my perception and connection with myself. It is really about our own connection with ourselves that improves self-understanding. Thus, we open a door to a better relationship with ourselves. I am able to be fully present with my patients and open to their current state of health in all aspects. We discuss together the core feelings that patients have about their health, symptoms, worries, fears, and aspirations.

We are able to better share the experience related to the doctoring with medications, labs, radiographs, and referrals with their unique contextual personal current state of health. We are able to discover the treatment plan relevant in their individual, unique, and personal lives and sort through the root cause of some of their health challenges. As a result, we doctor deeply in a very humanistic way that is connected to evidence-based medicine while highly personalized. We accept patients as they are and extend self-compassion. Patients love that."

Q: Why do you feel that Kelee meditation has helped you to enjoy your profession?

A: "Through detachment from the compartments of mental chatter of algorithms, pain, biases, and fears, I am better able to practice medicine that is patient-centered and rewarding. Both the patient and physician feel better in the process. My patients typically feel that they are clearer about their plan and just plain feel better walking out the door. The treatment plan is not a book algorithm, it is designed to fit into their relevant lives."

Q: So, in a few words, why do you enjoy your profession?

A: "My doctoring is deeply connected to the origins of my personal inspiration to choose a profession in medicine. With each patient and each day, I am able to feel meaning and help to bring my patients comfort. As I remain one-pointed in my greater Kelee, my feeling of self-understanding and self-acceptance is something that patients can sense. They often accept the feeling and leave the office feeling better. Often, I can help them physically through various treatments and interventions. But, in those circumstances where I cannot help them physically, I feel that I have extended peace from a non-linear mind."

Q: Spiritually, what does a physician experience?

A: "My light of awareness is shared with others from mental stillness to enable healing. I feel a sense of purpose. Healing has been shared. I feel like the patient has opened up and I have touched the patient with a vibratory rate of caring."

Q: Do you have any final words to share?

A: "After all, the origins of our name, physician, dates back to the early 13th century. Physician has been derived from old and modern French where "physicien" in French referred to a physicist and "fisique" referring to the practice of the "art of healing".
[https://www.dictionary.com/browse/physician; https://www.etymonline.com/word/physician]

Physician, my dear friend, be well and heal yourself first through Kelee meditation. It is by finding self-compassion and self-understanding that you will be able to share your mission to heal the world.

Basic Principles
of the Kelee Defined

The Conscious Awareness: a point of perception between the intellectual outside physical world and the inside world of emotion.

Brain Function: thinks, analyzes, stores intellectual knowledge, and runs the physical body.

Mind Function: mentally feels or senses as an objective observer and is synonymous with a relaxed sense of perception; thus mind function leads into deeper states of awareness and innate knowing.

The Surface of the Mind: a horizontal plane of electrochemical energy at eye level. A division point between the brain (or intellect) and deeper states of mind. These states are associated with inner contentment and an overall sense of calm.

Lesser Kelee: an electrochemical field of energy above the surface of the mind that moves out laterally from the center, up over the top of the brain, then down in between both hemispheres of the brain, and folds into the brain network. The energy in the lesser Kelee has to do with how one relates to the outside physical world—people, places, and things.

Greater Kelee: an electrochemical field of energy that flows below the surface of the mind, down to about where one's heart is and then turns upward to join the lesser Kelee at the surface of the mind. The energy in the greater Kelee has to do with how one feels about oneself on an emotional level. The energy of the greater Kelee is related to matters of the heart (i.e., caring, kindness, and gentleness).

Compartments: synonymous with "baggage," emotional "buttons," or "issues" manifesting as nonproductive, inefficient behavioral traits.

Looping: occurs when one's conscious awareness is attached to a negative compartment, resulting in a repetitive circulation of destructive thoughts.

Detachment from Internal Compartments: the space within one's Kelee, where one lives when one is unaffected by negative thoughts and emotions.

Processing of Compartments: the means by which internalized electrochemical negativity dissipates and dissolves. A result of relaxing one's conscious awareness, stilling one's mind, and detaching from compartments.

The Flow of the Kelee: when the electrochemical energy of how one thinks and the energy of how one feels flow together in unison without beginning or end. Within the flow of the Kelee is a single point of perception known as the conscious awareness.

The Anatomy of the Kelee®

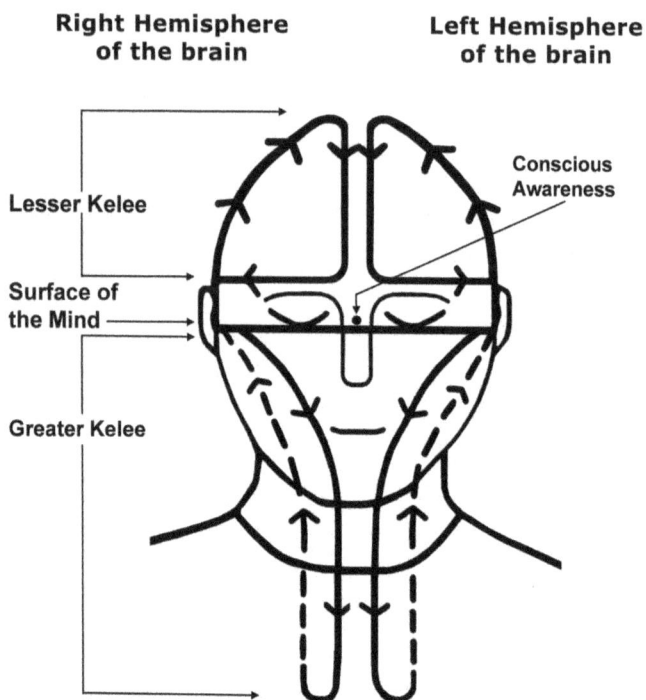

Right Hemisphere
of the brain

Left Hemisphere
of the brain

Lesser Kelee

Surface of
the Mind

Greater Kelee

Conscious
Awareness

How to Do
Kelee Meditation

Step One: *Approximately two minutes.*

Sit down, get comfortable, and begin relaxing brain activity. Mentally feel your conscious awareness at the top of your head and mentally relax this horizontal plane of awareness through both hemispheres of your brain, ultimately settling at the surface of the mind. At the surface of the mind, be consciously relaxed, but not thinking.

Step Two: *Approximately three minutes.*

After relaxing at the surface of the mind, mentally allow your conscious awareness to drop below the surface of the mind, to a still point within the greater Kelee. The goal is to let go of sense consciousness and experience total stillness for about three minutes.

Note: Before dropping from the surface of the mind into the greater Kelee, set your biological clock to come back to complete awareness in about three minutes.

Step Three: *Approximately five minutes.*

After experiencing stillness, return to full consciousness at the surface of the mind and reflect on what you noticed about your practice. Do not bolt into the day. The goal is to do Kelee meditation for ten minutes in the morning and evening to the best of your ability and get into the experience of life.

Recommendation: Keep a journal to record experiences and progress. One may think one will remember everything, but many subtle gems of wisdom and growth will be forgotten if not written down.

References

1. Rathbun, RW. Troubleshooting the Mind: Understanding the Basic Principles of the Kelee. Oceanside: Quiescence Publishing, 2010.

2. Lee D and Rathbun RW. The Kelee® Meditation Medical Study. Troubleshooting the Mind through Kelee Meditation: A Distinctive and Effective Therapeutic Intervention for Stress, Anxiety, and Depression. Oceanside: The Kelee Foundation, 2013.

3. Rathbun RW. Kelee Meditation: Free Your Mind. Oceanside: Quiescence Publishing, 2013.

4. Rathbun, RW. The Kelee: An Understanding of the Psychology of Spirituality, Oceanside: Quiescence Publishing, 2007.

www.ingramcontent.com/pod-product-compliance
Lightning Source LLC
Chambersburg PA
CBHW021608210326
41599CB00010B/657